SOMATIC EXERCISES FOR WEIGHT LOSS

Somatic Workouts for Everyday Wellness & Stress Relief

OLIVIA MORENO

CONTENTS

INTRODUCTION

Somatic exercises are mild movement patterns that alter your central nervous system to create new muscular habits. These new habits can mitigate chronic muscle spasms and discomfort caused by overuse patterns and other problematic musculoskeletal conditions.

Perform somatic exercises at home in a calm place while reclining on a mat or a dense carpet. Move methodically and mindfully and attempt to experience movement from the inside out.

Somatic Therapy refers to a body-centered/body-oriented therapeutic approach that utilizes the body's inherent ability to self-regulate, aimed at relieving and resolving stress disorders and enhancing the overall mind-body connection. It is anchored in the understanding that distress isn't solely a product of our minds but profoundly intertwined with our biochemistry.

Stress is a normal reaction to everyday pressures, but can become detrimental when it disrupts your day-to-day functioning. Critical/chronic stress occurs when people are unable to satisfy the expectations placed on them, resulting in bodily or psychological breakdown.

Our frenetic, modern existence causes most people to not pay attention to our internal senses (Interoception and Proprioception) and, as a result, neglect the interconnectedness of body and mind. However, it's within this very synergy that we can discover pathways to discharge pent-up emotions and nurture well-being.

This book will introduce various somatic exercises designed to delve into this profound mind-body connection. These simple yet potent techniques can help you navigate emotional obstructions, restore balance, and cultivate a more harmonious relationship with your own body.

Whether you're coping with chronic tension, or simply pursuing new methods to enhance your overall mental well-being, these exercises offer a transformative voyage into self-awareness and healing.

If you wish to reach into the deep crevices of your mind, remove yourself out of the mental cycle, regain balance, imbue yourself with optimism, and cultivate compassion

Benefits of Somatic Exercises

Absolutely, Somatic Exercises are indeed beneficial. They support the development of a more profound awareness of and connection with one's body, which promotes general wellbeing. Here's how:

Improved Mind-Body Connection

The purpose of somatic exercises is to improve your internal awareness of your body and its activities. Their focus on the body urges you to shift your awareness away from your mind and ideas and onto the feelings that arise inside your body. You may learn how the many components of your body work together and interact, as well as how your thoughts and emotions affect your physical body or specific areas of it, by concentrating on slow, deliberate movements. Your mental and emotional well-being is enhanced by this increased awareness, which forces you to face feelings and experiences that are stored in certain bodily areas.

Relaxation and Stress Relief

Stress is mostly caused by our overthinking and disorganized brains. Sometimes we need to shift our focus from our brains to our bodies in order to stop our racing thoughts, and this is where somatic exercises come into play. They use slow, methodical motions that may assist relax tension muscles and encourage sleep. They have a body-calming impact. Furthermore, the concentration needed to do these exercises offers a break from pressures, enabling your mind to relax and concentrate.

Enhanced Physical Well-being

Regular practice of Somatic Exercises can lead to enhanced flexibility, balance, and strength. The movements involved help to elongate tense muscles and strengthen weak ones, leading to improved posture and freedom of movement. This may eventually lower your chance of injury and improve your physical skills.

Emotional Release

Recent trauma research shows that we don't just experience emotions and distressing experiences in our minds – we also retain them in certain body regions. This explains how somatic exercises may be helpful in some way. They provide you the ability to explore and relieve tense emotional spots in your body. When emotions are experienced on a physiological level, they can be regulated through movement, trembling, or by paying attention to a particular body area. This can be particularly useful in increasing one's ability to regulate emotions, leading to enhanced emotional health and resilience.

Mindful Living

Finally, engaging in Somatic Exercises promotes a more conscious way of life. You become aware that you are more than your ideas of who you are when you establish a connection with your physical self. By emphasizing internal awareness, one may develop a more profound knowledge of themselves and adopt a more deliberate and attentive attitude to their everyday actions. This may improve your general well-being and quality of life.

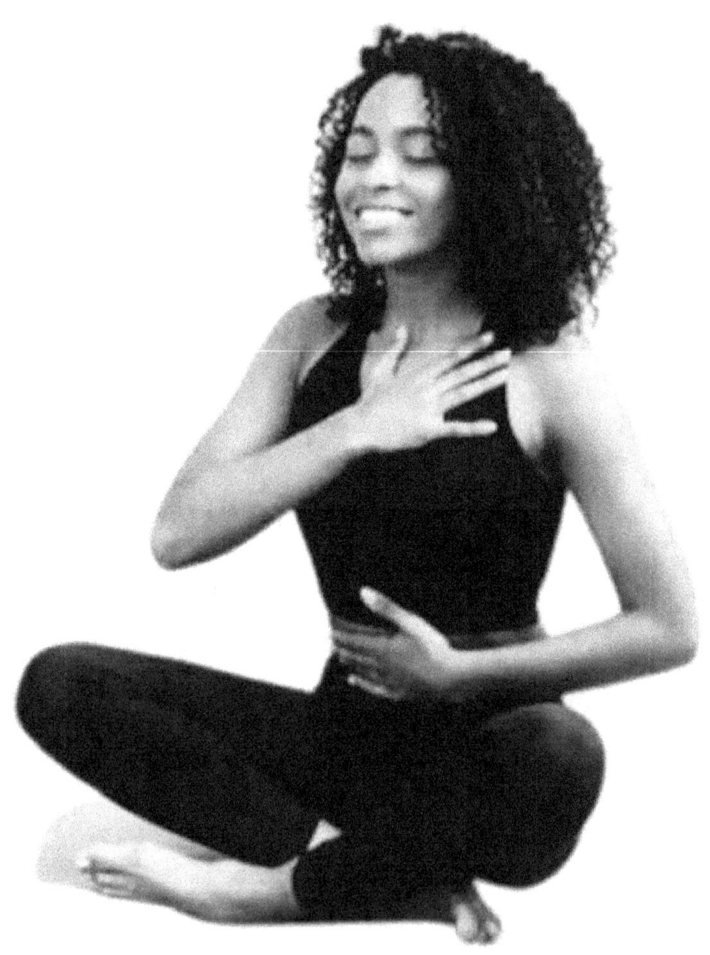

Somatic Yoga Meditation

Chapter 1

Types of Somatic Exercises

There are numerous sorts of Somatic Exercises, ranging from slow, focused motions to more advanced and hard positions. It is difficult to break down somatic exercises into particular difficulties since their goals frequently overlap. For example, a breathing exercise may assist in releasing anxiety, as well as processing trauma. That stated, the following are some popular forms of somatic exercises and their uses:

Somatic Exercises for Anxiety

Somatic Exercises for anxiety are meant to help manage and lessen symptoms of anxiety by increasing relaxation and creating a deeper connection with one's body. These exercises frequently entail deep breathing, grounding methods, and mindfulness activities. Examples include Diaphragmatic Breathing, Grounding, and Body Scanning.

Somatic Exercises for Trauma

These exercises attempt to help people address unresolved emotional difficulties held in the body as a consequence of experiencing a traumatic incident. Techniques such as Pendulation, which includes oscillating between tension and relaxation, may be very helpful. Other techniques include Progressive Muscle Relaxation and Somatic Yoga.

Somatic Exercises for Hips

Somatic Exercises for hips concentrate on enhancing hip mobility and relieving tension or pain in the hip region. These could include particular Somatic Yoga postures targeting the hips, Snail's Pace Stretching, and Comfortable Movements such as gentle hip circles.

Somatic Exercises for Anger

Anger – like any other emotion – does not merely happen in the brain. It also takes place in the body. Somatic Exercises for anger attempt to help people manage and express anger in a healthy manner, as well as better connect with those body areas that could retain experiences related to anger. These exercises frequently include releasing physical tension and cultivating attentive awareness of physiological sensations. The Voo Breath, Shaking Out Tension, and Progressive Muscle Relaxation are a few examples.

Somatic Exercises for Stress

Somatic Exercises for stress concentrate on triggering the body's relaxation response and minimizing physical indications of stress. Techniques like Diaphragmatic Breathing, Grounding, and Body Scanning may be very beneficial.

Somatic Exercises for Weight Loss

While Somatic Exercises alone may not contribute to weight reduction, rather they help weight loss attempts by developing body awareness, promoting movement efficiency, and lowering stress.

Somatic yoga, walking meditation, and gentle movement patterns are a few examples.

Somatic Practices

Becoming out of touch with who you are may happen more simply than many people would assume. When you're focused on external looks, the responsibilities of everyday life, and social expectations, your inner self might be disregarded. This is precisely what Thomas Hanna, a prominent somatic educator, underscored when he said: "Soma is the living body experienced from within."

Think of somatic techniques as a means of reconnecting with your body and tapping into its intrinsic knowledge. Somatic practices cover a number of approaches that incorporate attentive movement, breathwork, and body awareness.

Pioneers in the discipline came up with distinct systems such as the Feldenkrais method, Alexander technique, and body-mind centering, each of which provides a unique approach to somatic awareness and healing. By adding these activities to your health regimen, you may create a deeper sense of self-awareness, release muscular tension, improve posture, and lessen chronic pain.

Here's all you need to know about somatic practices and how you can utilize them for well-being.

What are Somatic Practices?

Somatic practices are a range of body-centered activities that assist people in reconnecting with their bodies to enhance health, well-being, and body awareness.

These practices are founded on the notion that the mind and body are not distinct entities but rather a unified system in which one part interacts with and impacts the other in significant ways.

Somatic practices comprise a number of approaches and exercises that concentrate on interior bodily sense and experience.

Rather than seeing the body as an object that is to be taught or fixed, these practices enable people to examine their interior sensations and movement patterns.

This entails listening to the body's signals, identifying areas of tension or pain, and utilizing mindful movement and breathwork to remove blockages and restore balance.

The ultimate objective is the growth of somatic awareness, which is a heightened understanding of the physical body and its interaction with the mind, space, and the world around it. Furthermore, it's about seeing the body as a source of knowledge and insight and a vehicle for personal development and change.

If you desire to delve into the deep corners of your mind, pull yourself out of the mental loop, recover equilibrium, inject yourself with optimism, and create compassion

What Are The 4 Somatic Practices?

Somatic-based therapy, somatic bodywork, somatic movement, and somatic breathwork are the four main kinds of somatic activities. In each of these categories, there are several distinct techniques and methods.

Somatic-based Therapy

Somatic-based treatment incorporates both physiological and psychological processes. It understands that our physical bodies and our thoughts are connected, with one impacting the other.

This method proposes that by connecting with our bodies, we may reveal deeper levels of our emotions, attitudes, and ideas. Examples of somatic techniques in this area include bioenergetics and Hakomi.

Bioenergetics (a therapeutic practice) includes integrating biological activities to ease physical strain associated with emotional discomfort. At the same time, Hakomi blends ideas of Eastern philosophy, especially Buddhism and Taoism, and other body-centric concepts such as mindfulness that employ bodily sensations, emotions, and thoughts to access and modify deeply established, unconscious patterns.

Somatic-based therapy may be especially effective in situations of trauma recovery as it releases painful feelings that are related to the traumatic experience and reduces cortisol levels.

Somatic Bodywork

Somatic bodywork comprises a spectrum of treatments that employ hands-on approaches to enhance physical function and promote well-being. Techniques such as massage, touch, and manipulation are utilized for relieving tension, increasing circulation, and restoring bodily equilibrium.

Specific practices in this category include Rolfing, a form of deep tissue bodywork that realigns the body's structural balance through muscle and fascia manipulation, and craniosacral therapy, which uses gentle touching to empower the client to recognize or release blockages or tension, particularly in the central nervous system, and improve overall health.

Somatic bodywork may be especially effective for stress management, with somatic exercises for stress being a crucial component.

Somatic Movement

The somatic movement encompasses activities that employ movement and sensory feeling to build bodily awareness, increase physical capability, and release stress. These exercises are commonly used in dance and performing arts for developing body flexibility, strength, and coordination.

Somatic movement practices include the Feldenkrais method, which employs gentle movements to improve body function and ease of movement, and the Alexander technique, which focuses on sensory awareness, self-perception, and conscious movement to teach people how to move more efficiently.

Somatic Breathwork

Somatic breathwork refers to activities that involve conscious and purposeful regulation of breathing to induce relaxation, regulate stress, and promote mental and physical health. Breathwork may have various health advantages, including reducing cortisol, the body's major stress hormone.

Examples of somatic breathwork include holotropic breathwork (HB), which employs regulated fast breathing to generate altered states of consciousness for self-exploration and healing, and transformational breathwork, which strives to integrate the physical, emotional, and spiritual elements of persons.

Incorporating these activities into your health regimen may result in significant rewards. For those who are interested, a plethora of information, including somatic exercises pdf, is accessible online to aid newcomers through the process.

Somatic Practice Technique

One example of a somatic practice approach is the fascial release technique (FRT). FRT entails employing slow, soft, and focused motions to release tension in the body's fascia or connective tissue to restore postural and functional integrity. This may help relieve discomfort and increase flexibility. It also helps stimulate the body's parasympathetic nervous system, which produces relaxation and decreases tension.

Let's now have a look at more strategies that come under the four categories outlined above.

Somatic-Based Therapy Practices

Emotional Freedom Technique (EFT)

EFT, which is frequently referred to as "tapping", involves self-stimulating particular acupressure sites while thinking about sensations of the body or uncomfortable thoughts/feelings.

It was invented by Gary Craig in the 1990s and is supposed to assist in minimizing negative emotional reactions and facilitate psychological recovery.

Eye Movement Desensitisation and Reprocessing (EMDR)

Developed by psychologist Francine Shapiro in 1987, EMDR is a psychotherapy that integrates components of somatic therapy. EMDR employs bilateral eye movement, touch, or auditory stimuli to assist in processing and making sense of unresolved traumatic memories.

Focusing

Focusing was established by Eugene Gendlin in the 1960s and is a person-centered treatment that includes paying attention to the "felt sense", a physical feeling that conveys crucial information about our emotions and what we must do in order to recover.

Reichian Therapy/Orgone Therapy

This treatment was established by Wilhelm Reich in the early 20th century and it focuses on releasing physical tensions that have been held in the body and are considered to be impeding the normal flow of life force, or "orgone".

Somatic Experiencing

Created by Peter Levine, this body-mind technique tries to release and resolve the "trapped" emotions that are associated with witnessing a traumatic experience by improving internal awareness (interoceptive, proprioceptive, and kinesthetic sensations) and fostering general well-being.

Tension and Trauma Releasing Exercises (TRE)

TRE was created by David Berceli and is a mind-body treatment that involves a series of exercises that are supposed to assist the body release underlying muscle patterns of stress and tension.

Somatic Bodywork Techniques

Body-Mind Centering

Bonnie Bainbridge Cohen established this approach that combines hands-on re-patterning of the body's structure, in addition to movement activities, as a way of achieving balance and encouraging a better knowledge of the body-mind relationship.

Bodywork and Somatic Education (BASE)

BASE was created by Dave Berger and is a hands-on method that employs touch, awareness, and movement to produce greater postural alignment and ease of mobility. It may also be coupled with psychotherapy for addressing painful memories.

Neurokinetic Therapy

Created by David Weinstock, neurokinetic therapy is a remedial movement technique that tackles the reasons for faulty movement patterns.

Rolfing Structural Integration

Developed by Ida P. Rolf in the 1940s, Rolfing is a method of hands-on bodywork and movement training that helps align the body's structure and improve posture and mobility via muscle and fascia manipulation.

Rosen Method Bodywork

This method was established by Marion Rosen and employs gentle, direct touch to assess muscular tension and encourage relaxation and emotional awareness.

Somatic Movement and Dance Practices

Alexander Technique

Founded by Frederick Matthias Alexander in the late 19th century, this approach helps retrain habitual patterns of movement to improve posture, decrease muscle tension, and boost general well-being.

Functional Integration (Feldenkrais Method)

The Feldenkrais technique was established by Moshe Feldenkrais in the mid-20th century with the purpose of strengthening the body-mind connection and total human functioning by developing self-awareness via elegant and efficient movement.

Awareness Through Movement (Feldenkrais Method)

In this exercise, students are directed through a series of motions to discover how their body moves and to enhance general function.

Contact Improvisation

Developed in the 1970s by Steve Paxton and others, contact improvisation is a dance style where points of physical contact offer the beginning point for exploration via movement improvisation.

Continuum Movement

Continuum movement was established by Emilie Conrad and is a dynamic style of meditation and movement therapy integrating sound, breath, and movement investigations.

Hanna Somatics

Developed by Thomas Hanna, this approach incorporates slow, deliberate motions to raise body awareness, improve motor control, and redefine the sense of physical self.

Skinner Releasing Technique

This technique was designed by Joan Skinner and blends imagery, movement, and hands-on companion studies to improve ease of movement, technical proficiency, and creative expression.

Somatic Expression

Jamie McHugh created this practice that integrates modern dance, massage, and mindfulness to foster body awareness and creativity.

If you've tried meditation in the past but were unable to complete a session due to distracting thoughts, uncontrollable urges, or intense emotions that surface as soon as you enter a state of stillness, it's likely because you didn't receive the proper instruction.

Somatic Breathwork Techniques

Conscious Connected Breathing (CCB)

This technique includes keeping a mindful, continuous breath, often in and out via the nose. The purpose of this deep, rhythmic breathing method is to foster awareness of the link between the body and mind and to induce relaxation and emotional release.

Biodynamic Breathwork

Developed by Giten Tonkov, the biodynamic breathwork and trauma release technique incorporates components of breathing, movement, music, touch, emotion, and meditation. It seeks to alleviate stress that is carried in the body and help people reconnect with their actual selves.

Rebirthing Breathwork

Founded by Leonard Orr, rebirthing breathwork includes linked and continuous breathing with no gap between inhaling and exhaling. The purpose of this is to relieve unconscious bodily and emotional stress, which leads to a heightened feeling of well-being.

Integrative Breathwork

This therapy approach involves breathing for accessing and exploring various states of consciousness.

It was established by Jacqueline A. Small and blends concepts from current consciousness research and transpersonal psychology. It may lead to great emotional release and spiritual progress.

Pranayama (Yogic Breath)

This is a traditional Indian technique that is centered on managing breathing to balance the body's energy flows. Pranayama exercises may vary widely in method, but all of them seek to promote physical and mental well-being.

Wim Hof Method

Developed by Wim Hof, dubbed "The Iceman", this approach employs breathing, cold treatment, and devotion to help you connect more profoundly with your body.

It incorporates a special breathing technique—similar to tummo (inner fire) meditation and pranayama—that attempts to activate the vagus nerve, boost oxygen in the blood and brain, decrease stress, and enhance physical performance.

The Wim Hof technique builds resilience by purposely pushing the body and mind to adapt to stressful circumstances.

Frequently Asked Questions

Is mindfulness a somatic practice?

Yes, mindfulness may be regarded to be a somatic practice. It entails developing awareness of the body, its feelings, and its movement, which are fundamental parts of somatic activities.

Is yoga a somatic therapy?

While yoga is not often classed as a somatic treatment, it has many features with somatic activities. Yoga fosters bodily awareness, intentional movement, and the link between mind and body. Some yoga practitioners also use somatic components in their practice.

What are the 5 channels of somatic experiencing?

Somatic experience® takes a 'bottom-up' method by employing five channels, or routes, via which the body may release 'trapped' emotions that are related to experiencing a traumatic event. These channels are sensation, imagery, behavior, emotion, and meaning.

How do you relieve anxiety somatically?

Somatic methods for anxiety release include mindful breathing exercises, guided body scans, progressive muscle relaxation (PMR), and embodied movement activities such as yoga or tai chi. These techniques help center the person, bring awareness to bodily sensations, and control the nervous system.

Somatic practices are strong tools for self-care, personal development, and better physical and mental well-being. Whether you want to develop your movement abilities or just alleviate stress, there is a somatic practice that may help you reach your objectives.

With the appropriate supervision from a trained practitioner, these techniques may be utilized to help you achieve new heights of health and vitality

Chapter 2

Somatic Meditation

A wandering mind might go in the way of obtaining a level of awareness, calm, and concentration that meditation offers. Most newcomers struggle to rein in their thoughts, frequently finding themselves trapped in a maze of anxieties, goals, or recollections.

Even with expertise, it's completely normal to find oneself battling with the problem of retaining attention.

Somatic meditation presents an innovative approach to this universal issue. It is a practice that stresses awareness of physical sensations and the perception of physiological experiences in the present moment as a way of enhancing the mind-body connection.

Research on this specific kind of meditation is not as comprehensive as it is with more traditional forms, but anecdotal (experience-based) data shows that this practice may be especially useful.

Research on mindfulness has revealed that it provides possible gains to stress management, emotional regulation, and general well-being.

Here's all you need to know about somatic meditation: its description, the advantages it gives, and how you may practice it.

What Is Somatic Meditation?

Somatic meditation is built on the idea that our bodies are not merely vehicles for our brains, but are intimately interwoven parts of our existence. In more traditional types of meditation, the emphasis is generally on the mind, with people aiming to reach a state of mental quiet.

However, somatic meditation reverses this paradigm, putting the body at the center of the practice. Instead of aiming to calm the mind directly, somatic meditation advocates a bottom-up approach where you tune into the physical sensations of your body.

Practitioners commonly integrate talk therapy, mind-body exercises, and physical approaches with somatic meditation.

These sensations might be as subtle as the feeling of your breath on the tip of your nose or as strong as the strain in your shoulders. By focusing attention on these bodily experiences, the mind may automatically quieten down.

This strategy is especially beneficial for boosting physical, emotional, and mental well-being.

Something tells us you frequently forget to put all the usual hustle and bustle on pause and just focus on yourself. It's time to sort up your priorities! Take a minute to heal, examine your feelings, center yourself, release all the pent-up tension, and rejuvenate.

What Are the Practices of Somatic Meditation?

There are various distinct techniques that come under the banner of somatic-based meditation, each of which is focused on growing awareness of physical sensations and experiences and enhancing the mind-body connection.

Body Scan Meditation

This technique derives from mindfulness-based stress reduction (MBSR) and entails deliberately focusing your attention on various regions of your body, from your toes to your head.

As you concentrate on each portion, you will detect any feelings that come, whether they're tension, warmth, tingling, or even the lack of sensation. This exercise builds a profound connection with your body by remaining present with and breathing into these feelings which may assist in bringing respite to our brains.

Breath Awareness Meditation

This exercise is centered on the experience of breathing. You concentrate on the physical feeling of breathing and expelling, observing how your chest, abdomen, and nose move with every breath. This strategy anchors you in the current moment and may help alleviate tension and anxiety.

Walking Meditation

Also known as Kinhin in Zen traditions, this practice comprises mindful walking when you concentrate on the feeling of your feet contacting the ground, the movement of your legs, and your balance. This style of meditation has been demonstrated to lower anxiety, sadness, and disease severity in Parkinson's disease.

Yoga Nidra

Sometimes referred to as 'yogic sleep', yoga nidra is a kind of guided somatic-based meditation that causes profound relaxation. You lay down and follow the guide's directions, often beginning with a body scan and then proceeding into deeper levels of relaxation and awareness.

The Benefits of Somatic Meditation

Somatic meditation provides a distinct set of advantages that distinguish it apart from more typical kinds of meditation.

This practice emphasizes the body's physical sensations and may give a more approachable road to mindfulness, especially for people who suffer from mental chatter during meditation.

Here are some advantages you may look forward to when you practice somatic meditation:

Enhanced Mind-Body Connection

Somatic meditation may generate an intimate dialog between your mind and body. By tuning into your bodily sensations, you will gain a better knowledge of your body's language, which results in a more harmonious mind-body interaction.

More Effective Trauma Management

When paired with other psychotherapies such as somatic experiencing therapy, somatic meditation has the potential to be a technique for processing and healing traumatic events that are carried in the body.

By concentrating on bodily sensations, somatic meditation aids with grounding, which enables people to slowly work through painful memories in a safe and measured way.

It is crucial to emphasize that without sufficient instruction, somatic meditation may be more of a stressor than a support for certain individuals, and result in re-traumatization. Therefore, if you have had a traumatic incident, you should seek the counsel of a competent therapist before you try somatic meditation.

Reduced Chance of Experiencing Stress and Anxiety. The introduction of somatic meditation for stress and anxiety might be a beneficial weapon in your mental health arsenal.

Somatic-based meditation such as yoga nidra helps modulate the fight or flight response, which is typically overactive in anxiety disorders and promotes calm and relaxation.

We address further low-impact techniques of treating stress and anxiety in our chair yoga for stress management post.

Improved Sleep

Somatic meditation for sleep creates a profound sensation of relaxation and aids the transition into a comfortable rest. By bringing awareness to the body and releasing pent-up tensions, somatic meditation may help establish the optimum circumstances for deep sleep.

Pain Reduction

Somatic meditation for pain harnesses the power of bodily awareness, which may transform your connection to pain, thereby lessening its severity. By concentrating on the body, somatic meditation may help you become more attentive to your pain feelings and work towards managing it more efficiently.

What to anticipate from a session of somatic meditation?

The following is how a normal somatic meditation session would go:

Find a Comfortable Position

Unlike other kinds of meditation, you are not obliged to sit in a cross-legged posture for somatic meditation. Instead, you should select a posture that helps you to be most conscious of your body. This may be **seated, lying down, or standing**. It's crucial that you feel comfortable and able to relax. Your hands may rest pleasantly on your lap or at your side.

Close Your Eyes and Start Breathing Deeply

Once you are seated, shut your eyes and start taking slow, deep breaths. Breathe in thoroughly through your nose and expel gently through your nose or mouth. Feel your stomach inflate like a balloon on an inhale then relax and let go as you exhale.

Scan Your Body

If you are distracted by noises in the room, just notice this and return your concentration back to your breathing. Start a leisurely scan of your body, beginning with your toes and progressing upwards. You may wish to wriggle your toes a bit and explore any feelings without judgment.

Pay attention to any feelings you experience along the way as you raise your focus up to your ankles, calves, knees, and thighs. This might be a sensation of relaxation, stress, discomfort, or even indifference.

Do not criticize or attempt to modify these experiences - just notice them. Slowly transfer your focus to the feelings in your lower back and pelvis, and then to your mid-back and upper back until you reach your head.

If your mind begins to wander, gently bring it back to the feelings of the region. Remember to keep breathing in and out as you proceed to the next section of your body.

Focus on Sensations

As you scan your body, you may notice specific feelings that are stronger than others. This might be a tightness in your chest, a tingling in your fingertips, or a heaviness in your legs. As soon as you find one, give it some attention. Again, do not strive to modify the experience, only notice and recognize its presence without judgment.

Integration

Once you have scanned your complete body, spend a few seconds just resting or sitting in stillness, which will enable your body and mind to digest the experience. Bring into your consciousness the top of your head down to the bottom of your toes. Feel the soothing rhythm of your breath as it flows through the body. You may perceive a sensation of tranquility, relaxation, or relief.

Return to the Physical World

When you feel ready, carefully bring your awareness back to the room. Take a full, deep breath, soaking in all the energy of this exercise before expelling completely. Wiggle your fingers and toes, stretch your arms and legs, and when you are ready, gently open your eyes.

During a somatic meditation session, you may experience a range of sensations and feelings. The goal is to watch them without judgment or opposition.

Over time, you may experience an expanded capacity to recognize subtle physiological sensations, a deeper feeling of connection with your body, and an overall improvement in mindfulness and well-being.

Following a somatic meditation session, it is usual to experience a sensation of serenity and relaxation. You may also find a better sense of connection with your body.

With persistent practice, somatic meditation may lead to long-term advantages such as increased sleep, lower anxiety, resolved traumatic memories, greater mind-body connection, and perhaps pain reduction.

Every individual's experience with somatic meditation is unique. The experiences, emotions, and advantages you experience may differ substantially from those of another individual.

This is perfectly natural and is a reflection of your unique body and thinking. It is advised that you begin somatic meditation with an open mind and ready to accept whatever comes your way.

It should be mentioned that without sufficient instruction, somatic meditation may be more of a stressor than a support for certain individuals, and this can trigger re-traumatization. Therefore, if you have had a traumatic incident, you should get help from a competent therapist before you try somatic meditation.

Can Somatic-Based Meditation Help with Trauma Healing?

People who seek out somatic therapy frequently have unresolved emotions that are connected to their experience of a traumatic incident. According to the American Psychological Association, the definition of trauma is an emotional reaction to a horrible occurrence such as an accident, rape, or natural catastrophe.

The traumatic incident might be a one-time occurrence, a lengthy sequence of events, or chronic, permanent stress. If trauma is not handled, this may lead to long-term repercussions, such as post-traumatic stress disorder (PTSD).

When practicing somatic meditation to release 'trapped' emotions that are tied to a traumatic incident, this should be supervised by a qualified therapist. The therapist may integrate somatic-based meditation methods with other psychotherapies in the session to assist in developing body awareness and release pent-up emotions.

Chapter 3

Somatic Exercises and How to do it

Diaphragmatic Breathing

This practice helps to stimulate your body's relaxation response. It requires deep breathing into the diaphragm rather than shallow breathing from your chest.

HOW TO DO IT

1. Lie down or sit comfortably.
2. Place one hand on your abdomen and the other on your chest.
3. Take a steady, deep breath through your nostril, allowing your abdomen to rise as you fill your lungs with oxygen. The hand on your chest must stay as motionless as possible.
4. Exhale gently out of your mouth or nose, allowing your belly to descend.
5. Repeat for many minutes.

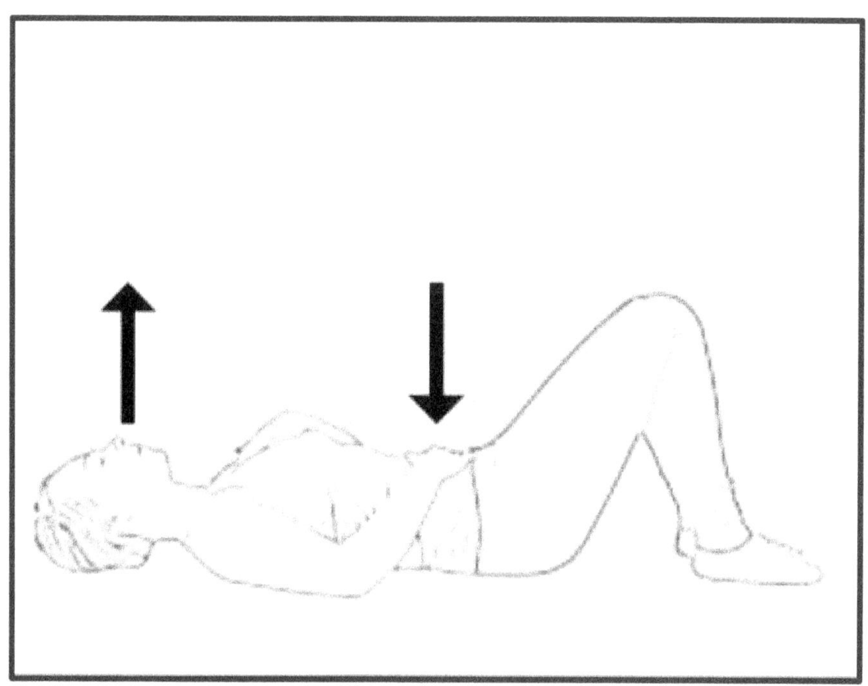

Diaphragmatic Breathing

Grounding

Grounding practices might help you feel more connected to your physical presence in the environment.

HOW TO DO IT

1. Stand up straight and feel your feet firmly anchored on the floor. Taking your shoes off for this workout may help you feel more comfortable.
2. Take a few deep breaths, concentrating on the feeling of your feet connecting with the soil.
3. Imagine roots spreading from your feet, attaching you to the ground as you feel linked to the earth
4. Start moving your weight from left to right, swinging like a tree.
5. Move your body weight from the front of your body to the back.
6. As you transfer your weight, bring awareness to your center of gravity, situated in the upper pelvic region and below the navel.
7. Bring your hands-on top of your lower tummy and sense your core.
8. Continue to sway from side to side and front and back while maintaining the hands-on top of your lower tummy.

Body Scanning

This approach creates heightened body awareness and may assist in detecting areas of stress or pain.

HOW TO DO IT

1. Lie down or sit comfortably.
2. Mentally scan your body from your toes to the head, noting any areas of tension or pain.
3. Spend a few seconds concentrating on each place and when you feel any tightness, breathe deeply and exhale allowing the area to relax.
4. When you feel the body part relax, you may go to the next one.
5. Continue this technique, until you reach your head.

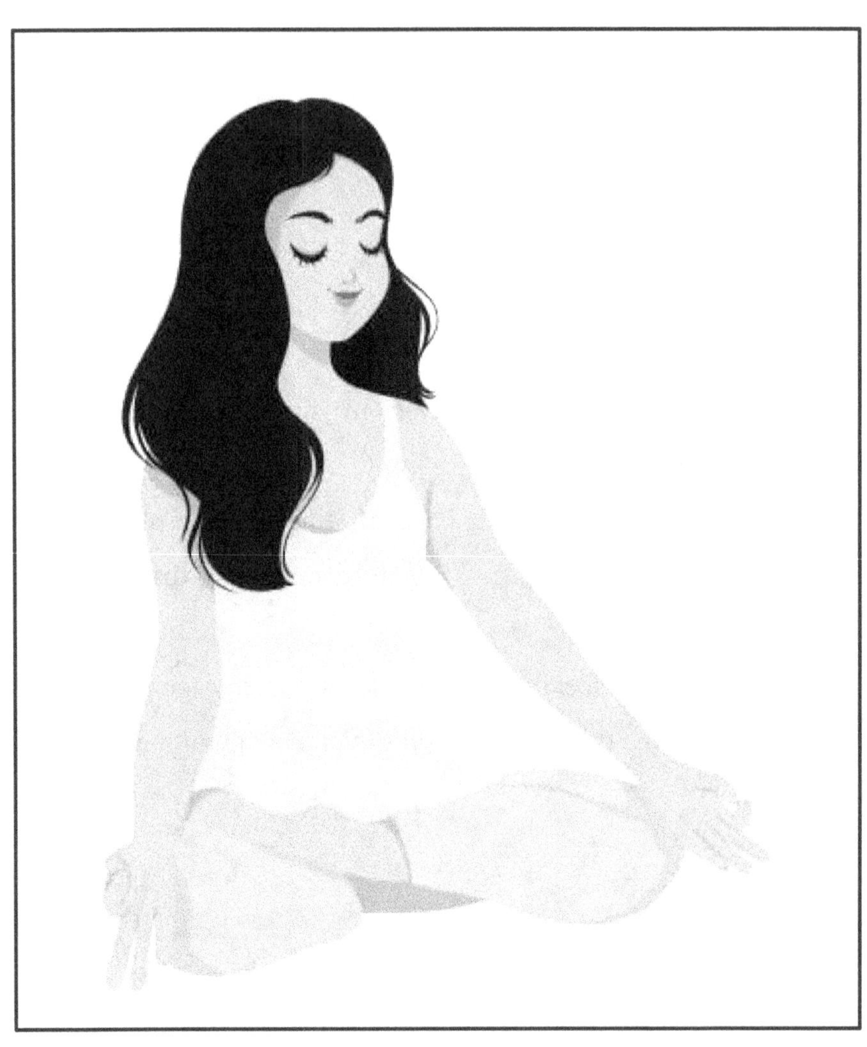

Sit comfortably

Somatic Yoga

Somatic Yoga includes executing classic yoga positions with heightened attention to interior physiological sensations. It should be performed with a trained somatic yoga teacher.

In somatic yoga, practitioners are encouraged to explore movements deliberately and with purpose, paying great attention to how each movement feels rather than trying for a certain end position. This strategy helps people to relieve tension, increase flexibility, and boost body awareness, which may generate a stronger knowledge of their physical and emotional experiences.

HOW TO DO IT

1. Choose a yoga position that you are comfortable with.
2. As you go into the posture, pay special attention to how each area of your body feels.
3. Hold the stance for a few breaths, continuing to keep awareness of your physiological feelings.

Walking Meditation

This kind of meditation mixes physical movement with mindfulness practice.

HOW TO DO IT

1. Begin walking at a leisurely, comfortable speed.
2. Pay attention to the feeling of your feet contacting the ground, the movement of your legs and arms, and your breathing.
3. If your mind wanders, gradually draw your focus back to the physical feeling of walking and restore your thoughts to the present moment.

Progressive Muscle Relaxation (PMR)

This method includes intentionally tensing and then releasing various muscle groups in the body to induce relaxation.

HOW TO DO IT

1. Commence at one extremity of your body, such as your toes.
2. Tense the muscles as firmly as you can for around 5 seconds.
3. Relax the muscles and experience the sense of release.
4. Continue to the next muscle group (like your legs), continuing the technique.

Sensory Awareness

This practice creates a heightened awareness of your sensory sensations.

HOW TO DO IT

1. Choose a quiet area to sit or lie down.
2. Close your eyes and inhale deeply many times.
3. Tune into your senses one by one, spending a few seconds concentrating on what you can hear, smell, feel, taste, and see (with your eyes closed).

The Voo Breath

This voice practice may assist in activating your vagus nerve, generating a sensation of peace and relaxation.

HOW TO DO IT

1. Situate an area where you feel comfortable and situate yourself in a comfortable position, either sitting on a chair or on the floor.
2. Bring your focus to your physiological feelings and to the current moment. Notice your breath in and out.
3. Take a big breath in.

4. As you exhale, create a "voo" sound, stretching out the vowel for as long as possible. You will feel this sound vibrate through your belly and chest.

5. Repeat numerous times.

Self-Hug

This calming activity may assist in easing emotions of discomfort.

HOW TO DO IT

1. Cross your right arm across your chest to feel your heartbeat, placing your left hand on your right shoulder.

2. Apply mild pressure and rock side to side.

3. Take slow, relaxing breaths while you hold this self-hug.

Shaking Out Tension

This exercise may assist in alleviating muscular tension and discharge extra energy that may have been created owing to stress.

HOW TO DO IT

1. Find a setting where you feel comfortable.
2. Stand up and start shaking your body, beginning with your hands and eventually including your arms, chest, and legs. Imagine you are brushing off dust or sand on your body.
3. Shake for a few minutes, then gently wind down. Bringing your body back to equilibrium.
4. Notice how your body feels after you've stopped shaking.

Washcloth

This is a full-body exercise that expands the shoulders, torso, and hips. You should feel as if you are wringing out a washcloth at your core.

HOW TO DO IT

1. First, lay down on your back and bend your legs so your feet are touching the ground.
2. Then, stretch out your arms to the sides. Point your right hand down and your left hand up.

3. Slowly roll your arms in opposing directions, so your right palm goes up and your left palm turns down. Rotate your arms further each time.

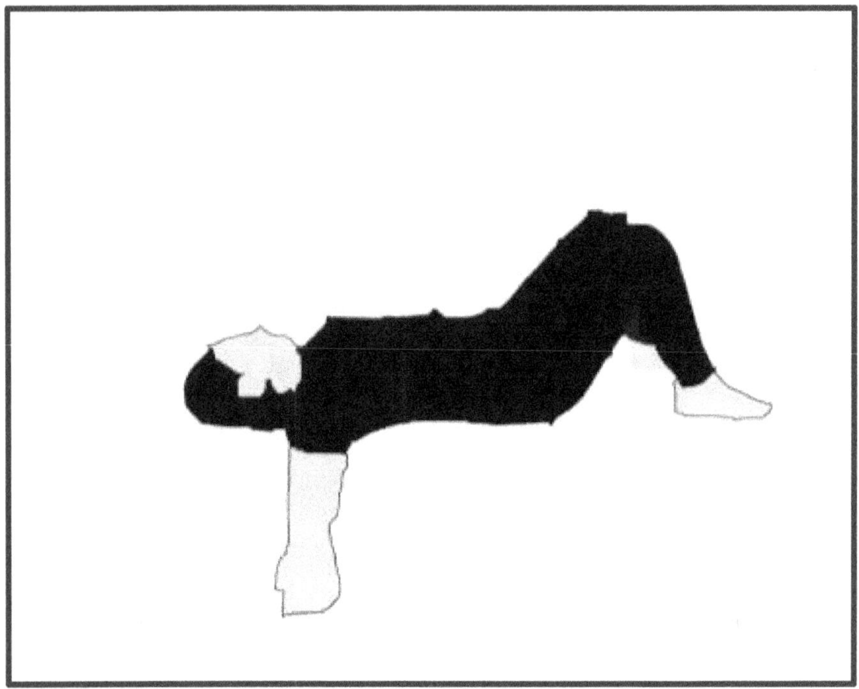

4. Make this a full-body action by integrating the legs. Moving in sync with the arms, drop your knees toward the palm-down side and move your head toward the palm-up side.

5. Repeat in the opposite way. Roll back and forth in a fluid motion like before.

6. Move carefully, watching how your coordination alters after repeating the whole exercise five to 10 times. Perform this sequence with your eyes closed to deepen the change in your body awareness.

Dancing

This fluid workout using simply the lower body stresses the link of movement in the legs and lower back.

HOW TO DO IT

1. Lie down on your back and stretch out your legs. Close your eyes and move your right leg to the side, making your lower back curve.
2. Then, move your leg back to the center, making your back flat.
3. Repeat this on both sides five times and see how it affects your lower back. After that, try moving both legs in and out like a pigeon toe and a duck foot.
4. Do this five times and notice when your back wants to curve or become flat. Let your back adjust in the right way.

Skiing

This exercise helps make sure both sides of your body are strong and balanced. It involves twisting your torso and back in a graceful way.

HOW TO DO IT

1. Bend your knees a little and turn your legs to the right and then to the left. Let your back bend and straighten in a natural way.

2. Do this movement five to 10 times on each side, and do it slowly and smoothly. Pay attention to how your back feels on both sides.

3. Stretch out your legs and try moving them in the same way, turning to each side five to 10 times. You might feel something in your back, but it won't be as strong.

4. Extend your legs long and attempt the same movement pattern, rotating five to 10 times to each side. The feelings in your back should be similar, but subtler.

Diagonal Arch and Curl

This movement pattern frees up your spine. Remain calm and comfortable while you perform it, never straining or crunching.

HOW TO DO IT

1. Lie on your back with your legs bent. Bring your left knee close to your tummy and hold it with your left hand.

2. Put your right hand at the back of your head (Place your right hand behind your head).

3. Exhale and stretch your spine as you raise your head to your left knee.

4. Inhale and arch your back as you drop your torso down. Repeat this action three times, then transfer to your other side.

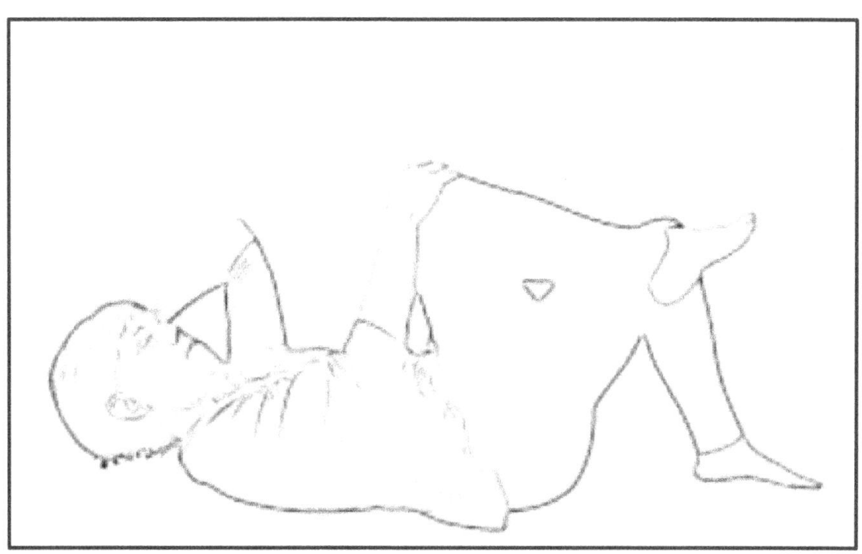

Diagonal Arch and Curl

Chapter 4

Somatic Exercise and Weight Loss

We all know that exercise is a critical component to losing extra pounds and boosting overall health, but what is the function of somatic exercise for weight loss?

In order to better comprehend this, it's vital to investigate all of the aspects that contribute to keeping a healthy weight and most notably, the causes that might be creating those obstinate extra pounds.

As we shall discuss further throughout this post, somatic exercises aid in balancing the nervous system and thus, it makes sense to start at the core cause of imbalance - stress.

HOW STRESS CAN LEAD TO WEIGHT GAIN

As exhausting as stress may be both intellectually and emotionally, it's vital to realize that stress also alters the body on a physiological level. When our body encounters stress, the nervous system shifts into a sympathetic, fight-or-flight state which stimulates the production of adrenaline and chemicals such as cortisol.

Research has repeatedly demonstrated that higher cortisol levels may stimulate appetite and induce desires for high-calorie, comfort foods. Moreover, cortisol stimulates the accumulation of fat, especially around the abdominal region.

When people feel stressed, they sometimes eat more food than they need to. This can make them gain weight. Stress can also make it hard for people to sleep well, which can make them feel hungry even when they're not. This can also make it harder for them to stay at a healthy weight.

All this to say, those obstinate extra pounds might be attributable to a little more than food and exercise alone. By opting to use stress management for weight reduction, you may be pleasantly surprised by the outcomes.

SOMATIC EXERCISES TO REDUCE STRESS

Somatic activities increase the mind-body connection. These specific exercises attempt to remove tension from the body, generate a feeling of safety and relaxation, and enable your nervous system to perform at its most ideal level. By participating in mindful movement each day, you're stimulating the parasympathetic nerve system, responsible for the body's "rest and digest" reaction.

It's not just about exercising, there's something deeper causing your weight issues that we need to figure out.

Somatic exercises go beyond only physical advantages; they give a gateway to understanding the fundamental causes of stress and weight concerns. Unlike standard training programs that may exclusively concentrate on burning calories, somatic exercises stimulate reflection and awareness of the body's feelings.

SOMATIC EXERCISES FOR WEIGHT LOSS

Because unresolved stress will always find a place to store itself in the body, the greatest thing we can do is identify it and develop a healthy outlet for stress via conscious breathwork, mindful movement, and additional somatic release work. In making this a regular habit, you may start to uncover the fundamental cause of your stress and establish a practical strategy for reducing it.

MINDSET AND WEIGHT MANAGEMENT

The mind plays a crucial influence in weight control. The thoughts and attitudes we have about our bodies may dramatically affect our habits related to food and exercise. However, seeking weight reduction by thinking alone can only go you so far.

This is because nearly 80% of the nerves in the body are afferent, which means they convey information from the body up to the brain. Only 20% of the neural system flows from the brain down to the body.

It may help to look at it this way: ideas are the language of the mind and emotions are the language of the body.

Although you may completely know the mathematics of losing weight in your head, it's likely your body is hanging onto unresolved sentiments about not being able to. This is where the power of afferent nerves comes into play and how somatic workouts for weight reduction may actually improve your outcomes.

CULTIVATING A POSITIVE BODY IMAGE WITH NERVOUS SYSTEM REGULATION

By now you know that somatic exercise plays a major function in nervous system control. A healthy neural system leads to wonderful advantages such as better mood, sustained quantities of energy, and a stronger sense of serenity and freedom in the body.

The more actively we engage in managing our neurological system, the more confident and self-aware we become. Nervous system modulation leads to higher self-esteem as well and may enable us to establish realistic weight reduction goals and nurture a more positive body image for ourselves. Although it might take some time to transcend those limiting ideas surrounding weight reduction, allow your body to lead you through what it takes to be successful.

Recall that although it might be easy, change is not always straightforward.

BENEFITS OF SOMATIC EXERCISES FOR WEIGHT LOSS

While cardio is crucial, including somatic activities into your regimen delivers extra weight reduction advantages:

Increase Metabolism

Even low-impact methods like yoga and Pilates may speed up your metabolism post-workout owing to the concentration on muscular activation. Your body keeps burning more calories for hours after a workout.

Build Muscle Mass

The mind-muscle connection you create with somatic exercises guarantees you engage your muscles from different perspectives. This shaping action may help replace fat with lean tissue for a leaner you.

Reduce Stress Levels

We all know stress leads to poor nutrition choices and fatigue — both enemies of weight reduction. Somatic activities soothe your body and mind, making them a beneficial stress-busting method

INCORPORATING SOMATIC EXERCISES INTO YOUR WEIGHT LOSS PLAN

If you're contemplating including somatic workouts into your weight reduction regimen, take some time to identify what works for you.

Somatic exercises do not need to be time-demanding. In fact, only a few minutes each day can considerably decrease stress and positively contribute to good weight control. Consider beginning your day with a somatic exercise or include a few of our recommended exercises below before or after a workout.

Here are three exercises that can help you lose weight and reach your goals.

The Cannon — Up- Take care of your body's control center.

The stress in this workout first triggers your body's natural 'fight or flight' reaction, releasing pent-up energy. The rhythm and steady breath then gradually pull you back into a still state, helping to relieve tension and restore balance.

How to perform it:

1. While standing up, inhale and extend your arms out wide to the side. Retain the breath while gently pressing the arms in, as if you were shutting a heavy door.
2. Then exhale deeply through the mouth, and release.

ENS Massage — Increase Interoception

The Enteric Nervous System, frequently termed the 'second brain', regulates digestion and influences mood. Massaging it may activate nerve endings, enhancing gut-brain connection and lowering stress.

How to do it:

1. Gently massage your abdomen in circles, beginning at the belly button and moving outward, concentrating on the feeling and rhythm.

Wall Presses — Down- Take care of your body and mind by controlling how you feel and behave.

Wall Presses enhance the proprioceptive system, improving bodily awareness and anchoring the neurological system. The pressure also releases serotonin, a 'feel-good' neurotransmitter, lowering tension and enhancing relaxation.

How to perform it:

1. Press firmly against the wall for a few seconds, then release and repeat, breathing as you push and inhaling as you release.

2. Keep your hands against the wall and concentrate on your breathing.

FAQS ABOUT SOMATIC EXERCISES FOR WEIGHT LOSS:

Do somatic exercises really work?

Yes, a large lot of evidence shows that somatic exercises may be useful in lowering stress, developing body awareness, and fostering positive body image. These elements all contribute to a comprehensive approach to weight control.

How long do somatic exercises take?

The length of somatic exercises might vary depending on daily and cumulative stress levels. Even 3-5 minutes a day might be effective.

How many somatic exercises should I perform each day?

When it comes to somatic exercises, we have discovered that depth over variety delivers the most significant outcomes. Our research advises picking 1-2 activities a day and repeating them as required until you've achieved a balanced condition.

While weight reduction may be accomplished in many different ways, it's vital to remember that lasting well-being and a good self-image are the ultimate aim. The mind-body connection plays a significant part in accomplishing our objectives and somatic exercises give a unique and very personal experience to your weight reduction journey.

By treating stress and weight problems from the underlying cause, which is, the status of your neurological system, you may greatly expedite your development and road to improved health and well-being.

Chapter 5

Somatic Release

Practicing somatic release comprises a series of exercises and strategies that help you reconnect with your body and release accumulated tension. Here's a basic approach to practicing somatic release:

Find a Calm Environment

Choose a peaceful, comfortable area where you won't be interrupted. This might be a tranquil area in your house, a pleasant outdoor spot, or any place where you feel comfortable and relaxed.

Movement

Incorporate moderate, focused movement into your practice. This might be stretching, yoga poses, or any other exercise that feels good to your body. Pay attention to how each action feels and let any emotions or feelings surface without judgment.

Rest and Reflect

After your practice, take a few minutes to recover and think about the experience. You could detect a sensation of relaxation, relief, or emotional release.

Regular Practice

Somatic release is most effective when done consistently. Try to set aside some time each day for this exercise, whether it's a few minutes in the morning, a break throughout your workday, or a relaxation practice before bed.

Recall that somatic release is an individual practice, meaning that each person's experience will be unique. It's crucial to go at your own speed and heed to your body's indications. If you anytime feel uncomfortable or uncertain throughout the practice, suspend the exercise and return to it once you are comfortable.

Also, if these sentiments or emotions are seriously harming your well-being, it may be good to seek support from a skilled somatic therapist or mental health professional for tailored guidance and treatments.

Frequently Asked Questions

What Are the Examples of Somatic Therapy?

Somatic therapy is a sort of body-centered treatment that tries to treat the full individual, including their mind, body, soul, and emotions. It involves diverse methods including massage, breathing exercises, and physical motions to assist release of pent-up stress held in the body, eventually facilitating healing and recovery.

Somatic Experiencing (SE) Therapy

According to SE, all human experience is preserved in the body. We do not simply endure trauma and stressful situations via emotions and ideas, but also through sensations that occur in our body. This style of treatment involves methods such as breath work, meditation, visualization, grounding, dancing, and sensory awareness practice. It needs to be supervised by a qualified therapist and is meant to help patients tap into their body's innate potential to heal.

Unlike other types of treatment, SE does not concentrate on thoughts or feelings (emotions) associated with the traumatic event and consequently does not immediately elicit unpleasant memories. Instead, it enables the individual to follow the feelings happening in their body to find their way to a sense of balance and calm.

Accelerated Experiential Dynamic Psychotherapy (AEDP)

AEDP is not primarily somatic therapy but uses somatic aspects as part of the therapeutic approach to assist patients in processing emotional events on a deeper level.

Dance/Movement Therapy (DMT) As the name implies, this kind of somatic therapy employs body movements and expressions as a therapeutic technique. It helps people to express themselves physically, explore emotions, relieve tension, and process experiences which may be especially good for those who find it difficult to put their thoughts into words.

Massage & Bodywork

Some kinds of somatic treatment include physical contact or manipulation of the body, such as massage. This may assist in alleviating bodily tension and encourage relaxation.

It's crucial to highlight that although massage and bodywork may be seen as types of somatic therapies, they are not a substitute for psychological therapy.

While they target bodily sensations and relaxation, they may not go deeply into psychological processing or treating trauma in the same way that other somatic treatments like Somatic Experiencing or Dance Movement Therapy could. Always talk with a skilled practitioner to establish which technique corresponds with your individual requirements and objectives.

Eye Movement Desensitization and Reprocessing (EMDR)

Although not a somatic treatment in the classic sense, EMDR is frequently described in the same category since it also understands the relationship between the body and mind.

This therapy practice helps reprocess traumatic memories by activating the right and left brain via bilateral eye movements or touch.

Is Yoga a kind of Somatic Exercise?

Yoga may actually be regarded as a Somatic Exercise since it focuses inward bodily awareness and experience. Somatic Yoga is not a separate type of yoga but rather a movement therapy, a technique of re-educating the way our brain detects and works the muscles.

Unlike certain yoga methods where the purpose is to reach a position, in somatic, the emphasis is the experience, skill, and ease of movement and transitions. This makes Somatic Yoga a moderate kind of exercise meant to aid us in releasing patterns of pain in the body.

While somatic yoga is connected with somatic principles, it is not a specialized therapeutic practice like certain other kinds of somatic therapy.

Is Walking Somatic Therapy?

Yes, walking may be an element of somatic therapy when it's done thoughtfully. This is commonly called as "Walking Meditation," where the emphasis is on the sense of movement and the touch of feet with the ground. It helps to link the body and mind, fostering awareness and relaxation, crucial features of somatic treatment.

Is Meditation a Somatic Exercise?

Yes, meditation may be called a Somatic Exercise when it incorporates a careful awareness of physical sensations, motions, or breath. Some kinds of meditation, such as mindfulness-based stress reduction (MBSR) and Mindfulness-based therapy (MBT) combine somatic concepts to produce a more comprehensive approach to promote overall mental well-being.

Is Mindfulness a Somatic Therapy?

Mindfulness may actually be considered a sort of somatic treatment. This is because mindfulness, particularly when practiced with a focus on physical sensations or movements, may assist in building a mind-body connection. It permits us to utilize our bodily reactions as a source of knowledge and healing.

Do Somatic Exercises Release Trauma?

Yes, somatic activities may aid in releasing trauma. However, this is an oversimplification of the process. In truth, somatic treatments assist the body in handling stress and tension held in particular physical areas, which promotes greater physiological safety. In turn, this assists with trauma processing and recovery. Somatic therapy, which incorporates a number of practices including breathing exercises, mindfulness, and body movement, might give opportunity for the body to regain its feeling of safety and return to a state of equilibrium.

This style of treatment focuses on the mind-body link and may be especially useful for persons struggling with trauma-related illnesses such as post-traumatic stress disorder (PTSD) or other psychological concerns such as anxiety, stress, complex grieving, etc.

Incorporating Somatic Exercises into your daily routine may be a transforming method to release pent-up emotions, decrease stress, and promote general well-being. These exercises provide a comprehensive approach to healing that treats both mind and body, enabling you to reconnect with yourself on a deeper level.

Chapter 6

Somatic Healing Techniques

Traumas dwell in your head and may also take a toll on your body. This might lead to bad feelings and disrupt your everyday life. Healing them is crucial for having a happy and healthy life. To do so, you might choose somatic healing approaches, which are recognized as being highly successful.

Before we describe how to practice these tactics, you need to grasp what they are. If you're seeking strategies to boost your mental and physical capabilities, this article may help you select the proper approach.

Somatic Experiencing (SE) Technique

This is a way of treating symptoms of trauma via therapy that was invented by Dr. Peter Levine. This therapy works by adding bodily movements and feelings into the treatment, resulting in the development of the body-mind link and letting the patient perceive their inner sensations.

Somatic therapy includes a patient recalling their painful memories, which may elicit emotional outbursts. However, before this step, the therapist will educate you about 'resourcing,' a strategy that may help you develop skills for managing these complicated emotions. Rather than concentrating on the mind, it employs a framework known as SIBAM (Sensation, Imagery, Behavior, Affect, and Meaning) that helps you concentrate on bodily sensations, develop body awareness, and find the 'tension places in the body' to process traumatic memories.

The basic idea of this treatment is the physical discharge of unresolved emotions since it is considered that such energies are predominantly imprisoned in the body. Research in 2017 also backs up this notion, since it revealed that somatic healing practices may help lessen the s PTSD and depression symptoms.

Running a never-ending rat race, burying trauma farther and further away, slipping into self-harming thinking patterns, living a life that's dominated by continual dread and fear – this is what an ordinary person goes through every day. Not confronting it will just drive you further into a negative spiral.

Trauma Stored in the Body

Trauma is usually retained in the hippocampus and amygdala in the brain's memory and emotional regions. Interestingly, these memories are related to the five senses: sight, smell, touch, taste, and sound. Your brain recalls what these senses feel to generate a visual representation of the trauma.

Traumatic memories, which are stored mostly in your brain, interfere substantially with how this function. This might lead to detrimental repercussions on your health. It implies that all these memories might show up in our body as muscular tension, headaches, stomach problems, etc.

Therefore, we may argue that when trauma is not completely processed, even in a normal setting, certain senses may remind us of the traumatic event, thereby prompting a fight-or-flight reaction.

How Do You Release Deep Emotional Pain?

It is usual to have diverse unfavorable experiences connected to life, profession, or relationships. Such encounters might eventually cause uncomfortable feelings that are challenging to bear. Therefore, many individuals hide their feelings so as not to be overwhelmed. Doing this will not help them overcome or move on from the terrible events. Instead, it causes these feelings to increase in their body over time. Gradually, these prior ordeals start to physically and emotionally affect the individual.

An unpleasant feeling that is ignored for too long may show as exhaustion, rage, unjustified animosity, or a lack of drive. Emotions that are not dealt with in a timely way may impair your relationships with others, physical health, posture, and even reflection.

You must reverse this so you may move on and let go of old unpleasant sentiments. All this emotional agony is produced by concealing these sentiments of the past. So, it would be great if you learned to regulate these feelings. This may be done in three main stages.

You might start by first identifying and admitting that feeling of yours. If it has been repressed for too long, you may have difficulties detecting it. However, this is a key phase, so you must comprehend and connect with the remaining feelings. You may seek the aid of a professional if you need to. According to research, the strength of a sensation might be minimized if you notice and describe it.

The second stage is to react to the feeling. The emotion stayed in your body owing to poor reaction. You need to work through the experience and waste the energy of the emotion. This may be done in numerous ways, depending on the degree and type of emotional suffering.

For example, you may practice journaling or speak it out. If the emotion is overpowering, it's advisable to undertake this exercise under the instruction of a skilled specialist. At the same time, you may treat it with somatic healing therapy. Intentional motions such as yoga, dancing, swimming, or martial arts might be done to relieve your body from the stored emotion.

The third phase is retaining the outcome of the work you have made in the previous two steps. It would be preferable to take charge of your body and practice self-care. Having repressed emotions suggests you have disregarded your body when it begged for attention.

Self-care may be simply performed via relaxation, meditation, and stress management. You might also explore nature and conduct soothing activities or somatic therapy techniques. In addition, you should make sure that you don't repress any feelings in the future.

Somatic Healing Techniques

As previously noted, somatic therapy follows the notion of increasing the link between the mind and body. It works via a 'body first' approach, which helps the brain experience and recognize every feeling and movement in the body. This is done via workouts and different sorts of treatment.

However, all somatic therapy activities are founded on basic somatic healing strategies. These approaches must be included in the somatic experience regardless of the method or strategy that is adopted. Techniques that are employed in a given treatment may vary based on the demands of the client.

The strategies that are used in somatic therapy include bodily awareness, grounding, and sequencing. Some of the somatic approaches are mentioned below:

Body Awareness

This is a foundational method that forms the cornerstone of any somatic healing treatment where tension in the body is handled to increase the body-mind connection. This approach helps to discover the stress points in the body where the unresolved emotions that are associated with experiencing a traumatic experience may be held. This is done simultaneously with some relaxing ideas to improve safety.

Titration and Pendulation

These two approaches, which are typically used combined, are among the greatest somatic healing treatments for the management of anxiety or PTSD symptoms. Titration is when the therapist assists you in working through a difficult memory one step at a time to prevent getting swallowed by the trauma. Any bodily change in feeling or movement is quickly observed, and the therapist will treat them as they occur.

This procedure is associated with pendulation so the patient will not feel uncomfortable. Pendulation is when the therapist helps you move between the stressful memory and a soothing condition when the distressing memory becomes too much to cope with. This helps build a rhythm and eventually releases pent-up emotions or sentiments that are tied to the memory.

This approach is used to soothe the customer. The therapist will ask you to recollect times, persons, relationships, and locations when you felt powerful and pleased. This permits you to recollect the resources that give you safety. During the session, the therapist will remind you to recall your emotional anchor if or when it gets overpowering as a method of fostering tranquility and safety.

What Does Releasing Trauma Feel Like?

Are you going through the inconvenience of somatic methods but don't know whether it's fruitful? You may check by observing the changes in your thinking or physiological feelings. These will tell you if you can release and resolve unresolved emotions.

Signs that you are releasing unresolved emotions include sometimes sobbing. This demonstrates that you can eliminate the repressed emotion and its enormous energy. Following a brief session of sobbing, you may feel considerably lighter, which signals the release of trapped emotions and trauma.

Trauma or repressed emotions may induce lethargy and tiredness and after they have been released, you may feel more energetic than before. You should also find it simpler to breathe, and each inhale and exhalation will gratify you. Also, you should feel energetic while you work out. Movements such as exercise, yoga, martial arts, and boxing can help you use the pent-up energy productively and make you feel terrific.

In addition, releasing repressed emotions and trauma can assist your physical health. Trauma and stress may adversely damage the immune system, therefore you may become ill less frequently after healing the trauma as your immune system improves.

Some Somatic Exercises for Beginners

Somatic exercises generally involve conscious activities that also assist in enhancing your mind-body connection. In this manner, you become more conscious of your physiological feelings and emotions. Therefore, it is good to conduct these somatic exercises for anxiety, sadness, tension, or the discharge of pent-up emotions.

These exercises alone cannot make up for the complete somatic therapy. They must be paired with the whole treatment session which includes counseling and other somatic healing procedures. These exercises may increase the efficacy of the treatment by relaxing the client and soothing and regulating their nervous system.

From the various examples of somatic exercises that are accessible, here are some that may prove to be helpful in your physically enduring therapy:

Healing Hands

Start by finding the stress place in your body. Place your palm over that spot and take long breaths. Your breaths should be slow and concentrated so you can feel the movement of your muscles underneath your hand. Continue until you feel calm.

Voo Breath

This is a simple, attentive breathwork for relaxation and calm. Start by breathing deeply until your lungs are full. Then, exhale gently while creating a low-pitched 'voo' sound. By doing this, you'll feel the vibration and movement of all muscles, notably the belly, chest, and neck.

Self-massage

This is not a difficult workout and merely includes gently massaging a stress region by stroking it with your hands in a gentle, circular motion. During this procedure, you'll feel the warmth and pressure of the hand.

Butterfly Hug

Cross your arms so your left palm is on your right shoulder and vice versa. Then, softly touch your shoulders with your fingers. Feel the movement of the fingers and the feeling of tapping on your shoulders. Make careful to take deep breaths simultaneously.

Diaphragmatic Breathing

Place one hand on your tummy and the other on your chest. Inhale deeply through your nose until your stomach rises more than your chest. Then, exhale gently through your mouth. Feel the sensation and movement of muscles under your hand.

Pursed-lips Breathing

Inhale regularly when sitting or lying down in a comfortable posture. Then, purse your lips as if ready to whistle or blow out a flame. Now, exhale gently through your mouth.

Box Breathing

This is a basic method for attentive breathwork. Inhale for 4 seconds. Hold your breath for 4 seconds. Exhale for 4 seconds. Simple, and it's done. Repeat this cycle a few times, experiencing the movement of muscles thoroughly every time.

The 5-4-3-2-1 Grounding Technique

This approach employs your five senses to bring you back to the present and control overwhelming sensations. See and notice five things. Touch four items and feel their texture, warmth, and everything. Locate and listen closely to three sounds and discriminate effectively between them. Locate two odors in the area. Finally, taste one item and feel it on your tongue.

Body Scan

This helps you identify the sections of your body that are under stress. Observe and ponder about how each body part feels. To execute this exercise:

1   Sit comfortably
2   Take a big breath in through the nose and out through the mouth
3   Close your eyes
4   Feel your body
5   Start at the top of your head Gently scan down through your body

6   Notice what feels pleasant or uncomfortable

7   Don't attempt to alter anything

8   Keep scanning down evenly

9   Notice each part of your body, all the way to your toes

A Mindful Walk

Walking in a calm atmosphere is one of the finest remedies. It will assist in quieting down your thoughts. However, the sort of surroundings influence when you take a stroll. It should be calm and you should be exposed to nature.

Running Cold and Warm Water on Your Hands

Run cold water for a few seconds and experience the feeling on your hand. Then run warm water. Feel the temperature change and how your hand responds to it.

Frequently Asked Questions

What is somatic shaking?

Somatic shaking is a way of relieving tension that is produced by trauma or stress. It achieves this by shaking the body to regulate the neurological system. The shaking helps relax the muscles and return the nervous system to its normal condition.

What are the hazards of somatic experiencing?

Dangers of somatic healing include re-traumatization, breaking down of barriers, and abusive contact. Due to the nature of therapy, the client is physically and emotionally exposed to the therapist. However, with the direction of a professional therapist, they may be prevented and controlled.

Is somatic healing real?

Somatic practitioners think that exercises and treatments that integrate the mind and body assist in relieving trauma and stress. There is some study and data, while limited, that supports this idea.

What does a somatic release feel like?

Somatic release makes you feel lighter, as if a weight has been lifted from you. You can breathe more freely and feel more energetic. Your sleep routine will also improve. Exercising will make you feel terrific and your entire physical health will also improve.

What are the critiques of somatic therapy?

Somatic therapy has been attacked for the lack of proof, which is not accurate, since there is a growing body of research confirming the efficacy of somatic treatment. Another issue is that unlicensed practitioners deliver somatic experiences.